# FEMDOM FOR NICE GIRLS

*A Self-Guided Manual for the*
## Caring Mistress

Lucy Fairbourne

Velluminous Press
www.velluminous.com

1.0

cover design by Holly Ollivander

# Femdom for Nice Girls

### A Self-Guided Manual for the
## Caring Mistress

Lucy Fairbourne

*This book provides guidance and reflection about a way of loving that includes safe and consensual discipline administered by a caring Mistress to her willing slave.*

*If you think you might be moving away from that, or are in doubt about the safety of anything you plan to do, you must not proceed until you have made sure your activity is safe, sane and consensual.*

# Table of Contents

# An Introduction for the Hesitant Mistress

*"See what strange arts necessity finds out"*

— Christopher Marlowe —
*Dido, Queen of Carthage*

"I'm sorry I've been such a chatterbox," Lucia said. "You know me: one glass of wine and I can't shut up!"

Jasmine kept her eyes firmly fixed on her glass of chablis. "No, no, it's my fault. I'm sorry if I seem a bit preoccupied."

Lucia knew that she'd been filling silences more than being a chatterbox. She waited for her friend to say something else, but Jasmine was silent.

"Everything okay between you and Jon?" Lucia persisted.

Jasmine shook her head and took a sip of wine.

"You haven't been fighting? I won't believe that, not you two."

"Not exactly," Jasmine said. "It's just that Jon seems to want different things than I do."

"I knew it! You feel ready to start a family, and he—"

"No, that's not it. Jon's told me he'd be happy for us to have kids. In fact, he'd be happy to do anything I want."

Lucia raised an eyebrow. "Seems ideal to me. What's the problem?"

"You don't understand. He'd be happy to do **anything** I want. "

The desserts arrived, and Lucia pitched her reply so that the departing waiter wouldn't overhear. The horrified way Jasmine had said, 'anything' told the experienced Lucia that her friend's problem required discretion. "He's made you an offer, hasn't he? Asked you for something? Something that he finds sexy and you find a bit … weird?"

Jasmine's expression was almost comical. "How on earth did you know?"

"Give me a moment." Lucia took out her phone and sent a text. A few seconds later the phone chimed and she read the reply. "Good, Cal's okay with me talking about it."

*"Talking about what? And why do you need his permission?"*

*"I don't need Cal's permission for anything." Lucia winked. "In fact, it's the other way around. I do respect him, though. I wouldn't share something like this if he asked me not to."*

*"Stop being so mysterious!"*

*Lucia scooped a spoonful of chocolate ice cream and let it melt in her mouth before continuing. "I don't think you have anything to worry about, once you understand what Jon's really asking. Knowing you both, knowing how you are together, I'd say you're in for the ride of your life." She savored another mouthful of ice cream, then leaned forward. "Listen, and I'll explain everything…"*

If you're the intended audience for this introduction, your husband or boyfriend has probably sprung a strange idea on you. He wants you to take charge of him, to take the dominant role in the relationship and particularly in the bedroom.

(If you're not the intended audience, feel free to stay and listen anyway, if you like).

It's easy to feel wrong-footed by such a request — one moment he's a regular guy who has your love and shares your life, the next he's telling you he wants to serve as your slave. If nothing else, it can all seem a bit sudden.

The process won't have been sudden for him. Chances are that the man who's just told you he wants to worship you, has been nervously rehearsing what to say for weeks while waiting for the right moment (and the courage!) to share this very private aspect of his nature with you.

The fact that he's managed to do so, shows that he really trusts you.

If you're now in a state of shock about this previously unsuspected aspect of him, or if you're simply worried that you won't be able to provide what he "expects", then try to put those concerns aside while you consider the following:

- The male desire to be controlled by a strong, loving female, is a common trait. It doesn't make that male is perverted, weak, broken, or less than a man; often it's the most successful, self-assured male who most craves the vulnerability of complete surrender when he's alone with his beloved woman.

- Accepting such a role does not mean you will end up responsible for some kind of "erotic domination service" designed to cater to his needs That's not what he wants. A submissive man is into servitude; he wants to be the one taking trouble to provide erotic (and other) services to you, not the other way around.

- Being in control of a willing male slave can open up all kinds of pleasurable possibilities. It means that his romantic and erotic attention can be a given — and available to you, in any way you choose to command.

- When you're in charge, all boundaries and comfort zones are yours to decide. Your needs, including your need to proceed at a pace that's comfortable for you, always come first.

- *Dominant You* will be his star-attraction; your commanding presence is more important than the details of what you do or command. If he wanted sexy commands to follow, why wouldn't he just find a list online and print it out? The thing that he wants cannot be printed out or otherwise counterfeited, because it's *Dominant You.*

To summarize: If you interpret your man's request for domination mainly as *you* having to do something naughty or nice for *him*, then not only are you placing unnecessary stress on yourself, you're headed to a place where you're not going to be able to give him what he needs in any case.

On the other hand, if you interpret it mainly as having the opportunity to make *him* do naughty and nice things for *you* to appreciate (and to have him love doing those things, and love you even more for permitting or "forcing" him to do them) then you have a lot less to worry about, and you'll be offering him the gift of servitude that he craves.

Of course, your man has expectations too. If the only thing you ever demanded of your "slave" was to be your regular chick-flick date, then he'd surely be disappointed, because...

> *The power of female dominance can satisfy a male's submissive needs but it can't make them go away.*

Submissive needs are deep-rooted, possibly going all the way back to childhood, and the submissive male has no way to shrug them off. Your man's choices were to seek solace with a secret fantasy life (or worse) or to be open with you — and given that you're reading this, it seems he did the decent thing.

So, as a caring Mistress you'll want to meet those needs — in a way that's good for you, and good for him.

In that order.

A word of warning: it's possible that a man who self-identifies as sub-missive, is really only interested in having you help act out his scripted fantasies. This is the kind of man who turns up at the bedroom door knowing exactly what he wants...

> *"Tie me up. Spank me. Not hard enough. That's better. Now untie me.*
> *Command me to kneel.*
> *Now make me go down on you."*

...except there's no need for him to say any of this, because the dominatrix in his fantasy understands (telepathically, I guess) exactly how he expects to be "dominated".

Such a deceitful scenario cannot lead to a mutually satisfying erotic encounter. At best you'll be left bewildered, at worst you'll feel like a failure because you weren't telepathic enough to "dominate him properly". The existence of men like this may explain some of the female hesitance about taking on sexually dominant roles in the first place.

Anyway, that kind of pretence is not what this book is about. A man who truly and unselfishly wishes to serve you might hope desperately that you will take pity and spank him, he might yearn to be permitted to please you with his mouth, but he will never expect or demand these things, or blame you when they don't happen. Instead, he will want them only once you're ready, when you want them too.

In turn, as a caring Mistress you *will* be interested in fulfilling his needs, though not according to his schedule or agenda — or even in the way he expects. You'll make some things happen for purely selfish reasons, and you'll probably allow other things to happen as your unselfish gift to the man you love. Eventually, you might find you come to enjoy the second kind of thing more than you ever expected; doing consensual sexy stuff with a loving partner can have that effect.

The important thing *for both of you* is that you get to decide on both the menu and timing, not him.

By now, I hope you understand that there's no need for you to try to conform to the stereotypical male-fantasy image of the bitchy, corseted dominatrix with her fetish shoes and her riding crop. My advice is *not* to conform to that image — unless you come to actively wish it yourself. Your submissive male partner might think he needs you to be leather-clad Miss Whiplash, but what he really needs is to be erotically persuaded that you value him highly enough to wish to own him and use him as your personal slave.

So, it really doesn't have to be all about leather and spike heels.

It does have to be about understanding your own needs — and your responses to your man's needs. It might also be about helping him understand his *real* needs, instead of the needs he's come to believe he has. And of course, it has to be about honest communication.

Mainly, though, it has to be … *as you wish.*

# *Guidance on the Workbook Sections*

At the end of each main chapter in this book is a "guided journal" section designed to help you to clarify your immediate responses and explore your attitudes to the subjects discussed. As you fill these in, bear in mind that…

### There Are no Right Answers!

…there are only *your* answers.

Your slave might well be curious to know what you write in these sections, but you should not allow him to do so.

Knowledge is power, and the only power your slave needs within your shared fantasy of domination and submission, is the power to please you. He can get this from his own knowledge of you, and from the instructions, guidance and feedback you offer.

Empowering him further by sharing the private feelings and thoughts that you will explore in this Workbook, would be counter-productive to a part of your relationship with him that can only be based on an *imbalance* of power.

Please don't feel pressured to answer any set of questions in one sitting. Some parts may require a period of personal reflection, or even a frank discussion with your slave. Take all the time you need to think about what you want, how you are going to benefit, and how both of you are going to gain pleasure and satisfaction from the shared fantasy you are creating together.

# *Boons*

"Boon: That which is asked or granted as a benefit or favor;
a gift; a benefaction; a grant; a present."

*Webster's Revised Unabridged Dictionary*

A boon is a favor granted by a superior to an inferior. To you, as a Mistress who owns and cares for a submissive male, it means setting aside a period of time with your slave, during which you will accept his submission and gift him with your dominance.

Granting your slave a boon generally means that you and he will mentally enter "Mistress space" where you will engage in some female-led erotic (or at least, eroticized) activity. The boon is always at your discretion, so your slave can never be sure when the next one will happen. When you do grant a boon, he will experience it with the maximum possible intensity, and then remember it long after it is over — perhaps for the rest of his life. He will also have no expectation that it will be repeated any time soon; by its nature, a boon is a rare prize, offered or withheld at your whim and received gratefully by your slave. The slave's inability to be sure of winning that prize is an important part of what makes it so precious to him.

So, never allow your slave to lose sight of the fact that boons are yours to bestow and never to be demanded as his right. Such confusion is not helpful to him, or to you.

If you enjoy a given boon enough to indulge your slave with it regularly, he might get into the habit of expecting it. Always remain clear that you have the right to suspend the boon whenever you like, or even to withdraw it entirely. Your slave will not like this possibility but he would like the alternative even less: to have the activity at *his* discretion could only mean that he, rather than Mistress, is in control.

Thinking about female-led erotic activities as boons, and assigning them a different mental space ("Mistress space"), naturally separates them from other aspects of your lives, areas where you need your man to be strong, independent and resourceful.

It also establishes the important principle that Mistress space, where he is able to express and explore his submissive nature with you, can only exist if you are fully in charge of everything including the boundaries of Mistress space itself.

The boons most desired by a submissive male will usually be those that deepen his feeling of being enslaved by his Mistress through one or more of the following:

- Physical Punishment
  Any activity whose main purpose is to cause erotic pain or discomfort to the slave.

- Erotic Servitude and Sacrifice
  Any activity where the slave foregoes his potential pleasure or comfort in favour of yours.

- Degradation of Status
  Any activity that strips away your slave's normal standing and demonstrates his lowly status as your property.

- Verbal Humiliation
  Any speech that aggressively belittles your slave or undermine his sense of self-worth.

The fourth item, verbal humiliation, can be seen as a kind of "edge play". It is risky because its power comes from attacking the slave's sense of self-worth. Your slave might well get off on this, but you should not indulge him unless you are quite certain he is not vulnerable to such treatment. The denial of his manhood that he finds arousing tonight, might mortify him tomorrow. The section on *Degradation vs Humiliation* on page 66 goes into more detail on this matter.

The other three items are not aimed at the slave's sense of self-worth (instead they address his physical body and his status) so they do not carry the same risk. All three have some cross-over. For example, if you present the boon of a beating as something your slave is being asked to "take for Mistress" then the physical punishment of the whip blurs into a sacrifice of pain endured; if you grip the collar that is a symbol of control and restraint, and use it to direct his mouth toward your pussy, then servitude blurs with degradation.

Here are several types of treatment that a typical slave might hope to receive as part or all of a boon, depending on his personal kinks and situation:

- to be spanked, paddled or whipped
- to be made to present himself vulnerably naked, while you remain dressed.
- to be reduced to the status of an animal by being made to go on all fours or to wear a collar
- to be tormented with ice cubes or drops of hot candle wax
- to be interrogated and forced to confess to some imaginary or trivial wrongdoing
- to be permitted to worship your entire body
- to be permitted to worship your pussy
- to see you wearing fetish costumes or footwear
- to be made to perform menial household chores while naked or otherwise degraded
- to play a rigged board or card game with you that involves unpleasant or painful forfeits when he loses
- to kneel before you and give you a pedicure
- to receive constructive, loving criticism/training
- to be forced to wear sexy female clothes
- to have his penis teased without being permitted to come
- to be "forcibly" penetrated by you with a dildo or strap-on
- to be permitted to bring you to orgasm through intercourse
- to be permitted to have an orgasm himself
- to play out a detailed role-play fantasy with you (see *Ritual and Role-Play* on page 63 for more discussion of this and several possible examples).

A boon might be an elaborate scene complete with props, rituals and stage-directions that you provide for your slave, but it can also be straightforward and trouble-free. Your slave will certainly fantasize about the showy, time-consuming kind but he will also take satisfaction from a simple boon that gives him what he craves most: your erotic, dominant attention.

For example, if you grant him the boon of being kept naked and reposing at your feet while you watch a movie together, then you are fitting the main part of the boon alongside a regular activity that you might well do as a couple anyway. The main differences are that he's a little less comfortable, and that you have more space on the couch. Maybe you'll arrange an "intermission" in which you send him to the kitchen to bring you refreshments.

A typical submissive male will enjoy the degradation and servitude described in this boon, but he will also long for his Mistress to be more overtly sexual with him. With this in mind, you may choose to include some erotic contact that will please both of you. In the previous example, you could order a foot massage as you watch the movie together. Later, you might complete the boon with a physical punishment or by permitting him to worship you orally.

While a boon might include any number of orgasms, none of them need to be his. There is no reason for any boon to include sexual release for your slave. If you have decided to subject your slave to a regime of male chastity (see the chapter *Orgasm Control* on page 79 for more information), then a boon that includes male ejaculation may well be the exception rather than the rule.

As a caring Mistress you will naturally wish to grant boons that satisfy your slave's needs, but don't forget that his deepest need is to please and serve you, so don't feel shy about granting boons chiefly or solely for your own pleasure. Even if they don't scratch your slave's immediate submissive itch, they remain boons.

One of his deepest sexual needs is to sacrifice on your behalf; this man is your slave — he is desperate to be your slave. Lovingly pushing his boundaries is a way of helping him to grow and explore, and the experience of pleasing you (and hearing you confirm that he has done so) is its own erotic reward.

## *Quickie Boons*

A quickie boon is a piece of dominant play that you allow to strike on a whim and that takes only a few moments. It should be something that's fun for you and that demonstrates or enhances your control over your slave.

If you ever use a quickie boon to provide an instant reward when your slave has done something particularly pleasing, keep things unpredictable enough to prevent him getting the impression that it is something he can earn whenever he likes. If he learns the habit that a "good deed" always leads to a quickie boon, then he may believe himself able to trade good behavior for dominant rewards; such a false belief is not helpful to him.

As with any boon, the quickie boon does not have to be directly pleasing for your slave. The idea is that you go from normal life, into the quickie boon, and back out again perhaps within seconds, or at most a few minutes.

Examples of quickie boons:

- A fleeting grope to arouse him while letting him know in no uncertain terms that his genitals are your property.
- Having him bare his rump for just long enough to allow three paddle or crop strokes, after which he pulls his pants up and you both continue as normal.
- Grabbing him forcefully and pulling him in for a long kiss.
- As above, but instead of pulling him into a mouth-kiss, guiding him down to perform a "quickie" cunnilingus on you.

As you see, while the activity of the quickie boon is erotic, it doesn't have to be kinky in itself. The important things are that the slave understands that you have favored him by pulling him into Mistress space where he has the benefit of your dominant attention for a moment; and that like any other boon it is entirely at your discretion.

### *Slave-Requested Boons*

The definition at the beginning of this chapter states that a boon is something that can be "asked or granted", and the old stories are full of knights and heroes begging their rulers for boons. Of course, the rulers were empowered to decide whether to grant the requested boon (and whether to allow such requests in the first place); the same goes for you.

Why might you permit or even encourage your slave to request a boon? The most important reason may be the pleasure you can take in having him express his submissive desire for you. Another reason might be that you want to find out something he wants deeply, so that you have the choice of giving it to him.

However, since your slave gets off on reducing his own power and enhancing yours, his natural preference might be to leave all questions of boons in your hands; he might find it very difficult to express his own desires to you. If so, and if you want to hear him beg for it, motivate him. Give him permission to ask, and let him know when such requests are appropriate and how they should be made. If you like, let him know that if he doesn't appear enthusiastic enough about boons, you won't bother with them either. In saying this you would not be withdrawing your female dominance, but expressing it even more deeply.

A slave who understands the nature of boons, will not need to be told to avoid overloading you with requests for his own benefit. Instead, his prime motivation should be that he thinks you will enjoy the request. And of course, he will understand that being allowed to request a boon, is not the same as being allowed the boon.

You can also choose to permit only certain kinds of boon; for example if you have taken control of his orgasms, that control will be less perfect if he thinks he has a chance to persuade you to caress his penis for a while, or maybe even to wheedle his way into an orgasm. Make your slave understand that nagging and illicit requests will have the opposite effect to the one he desires. His submission and service to you is *not* an investment that entitles him to some kind of guaranteed return, nor is it a deposit in the "sexual favors bank" that he can withdraw on demand later.

A final spin on the slave-requested boon is where you offer your slave a choice of boons and instruct him to pick one. As before, he might try to push the responsibility back to you on the grounds that a "true submissive" should not have the power to choose. That's nonsense, of course; a true submissive should choose when he's told to choose.

If you need to correct this tendency, you can force his hand by placing a time-limit after which the offer of the boon will be withdrawn altogether. Enjoy watching him squirm, struggling to choose as the time runs down, and feel free to reject his choice and substitute an alternative boon, if you decide that's appropriate. That way, you can force him to accept your authority twice: first when he obeys you in choosing for himself, and secondly when he ends up getting what you choose anyway.

# *Reflecting on Boons*

This section is for you to draw together your thoughts and to clarify your feelings about the boons that you might grant to your slave.

Three boons that I can enjoy together with my slave:

1. _____

2. _____

3. _____

Three boons that are neutral for me, but that I think would appeal to my slave:

1. _____

2. _____

3. _____

I'd consider granting a boon that was merely neutral for me    Yes ☐

   No ☐

Three boons outside my comfort zone but that I think would appeal to my slave:

1. _____

2. _____

3 _____

I'd consider granting a boon outside my comfort zone

Yes ☐
No ☐

I think my slave could enjoy a boon that was
too far out of my comfort zone for me to enjoy

Yes ☐
No ☐

It might be good to expand my horizons by sometimes
granting a boon slightly outside my comfort zone

Yes ☐
No ☐

Three boons that I would enjoy but that are outside my slave's comfort
zone:

1. _____

2. _____

3. _____

I'd consider granting a boon I'd enjoy

Yes ☐

but that was outside my slave's comfort zone:

No ☐

It would be good to expand my slave's horizons

Yes ☐

by granting boons outside his comfort zone:

No ☐

Some implications of my answers about my own comfort zones:

_____

_____

_____

_____

_____

_____

Some implications of my answers about my slave's comfort zones:

_____

_____

_____

_____

_____

_____

I would consider granting my slave a boon when:

_____

_____

_____

_____

_____

_____

I will restrict the boons I allow my slave as follows:

_____

_____

_____

_____

_____

_____

If my slave pressured me to grant more/different boons, I would:

_____

_____

_____

_____

_____

_____

The benefits I will receive from granting boons include:

_____

_____

_____

_____

_____

_____

The benefits my slave will receive from my boons include:

_____

_____

_____

_____

_____

_____

_____

I would sometimes permit my slave to request boons:     Yes ☐

No ☐

Some advantages of my previous choice are:

_____

_____

_____

_____

_____

_____

Some disadvantages of my previous choice are:

_____

_____

_____

_____

_____

_____

I could overcome some of those disadvantages by:

_____

_____

_____

_____

_____

_____

# Quests and Tasks

"Anon he rode unto the pavilions, and saw the lady that was his quest"

— Sir Thomas Mallory —
*Le Morte d'Arthur*

In ancient Rome or Greece, back in the days when real slavery was a widespread fact of life, the main advantage of owning a slave must have been that the wealthy Roman or Greek citizen could set the slave to work. Various slaves would have spent their time laboring in the fields, running errands, chopping wood, caring for the domestic animals, preparing meals, or cleaning the villa. Particularly prized were those who were highly educated, since they would fill more valuable roles by serving as secretaries and scribes, even as teachers or doctors.

Most of the people on the receiving end of this forced-labor scheme probably worked grudgingly and only under threat of violent punishment, but your slave will serve you willingly and gratefully as long as he is made to feel that your commands are expressions of your dominance, and that the outcome being demanded of him is something that you need or value.

Of course, if your slave runs an errand then you'll probably value the fact that you have one thing less to do, but I'm talking about something a little more subtle than that. It's the difference between:

1. *"Honey, I want you to cook tomorrow night, I'm not going to have time."*

2. *"Honey, I want you to cook tomorrow night, I've been craving one of your home made burgers."*

3. *"Honey, I want you to cook tomorrow night so I can spend more time with our guests."*

The first request is a reasonable one: you are short of time, so you ask your slave to do the cooking.

If your intention is to make this part of a dominance game, however, you haven't given your slave much to hang his submission on. What tangible benefit will you receive by having this extra free time? If your slave fails the task, will you suffer somehow? And by extension, if he succeeds is he protecting you from possible suffering? Your slave has no way of knowing.

In the second and third cases, you are demanding that he satisfies a couple of very specific requirements: enjoying the home-made hamburger that you crave, or having the leisure to participate in a social gathering that's important to you. If he fails, you will miss out on these rewards. This sense that there is something important at stake for you *and that you are relying on him to provide it*, is what engages your slave's submissive, service-oriented side with the task at hand.

In case there's any doubt, your slave has no business refusing or grumbling because you "just" used him to save some of your time. I made up these examples solely to demonstrate how the slave finds his servitude to you more emotionally and erotically fulfilling, if he can believe (even if only within the fantasy you're creating together) that you have a real need or desire for whatever it is that he's been instructed to do, and that you value and appreciate his efforts in completing it.

As well as hoping to earn your approval, your slave will probably be alive to the possibility that he might *fail* to meet your needs, and will do his best to ensure that does not happen. The *frisson* of unease he feels at the possibility of you being disappointed in him, may well be a big part of the submissive excitement he feels at being given a Quest or Task in the first place.

## Quests Are Not the Same as Boons

At first sight you might think that a Quest or a Task is just another kind of boon, but there's an important difference: the boons from the previous chapter were openly and physically erotic. They involved you and your slave in pleasurable and painful activities like foot rubs, whippings and cunnilingus.

Commanding your slave to depart on a Quest to pick up some meat and potatoes from the grocery store is unlikely to include such things. Instead, your slave's submissive response will be of the mental kind, purely inside his head as he goes around the shelves and chiller units, hoping to bring you the exact kinds of meat and potatoes that you will find satisfactory — and worrying that he might somehow get it wrong.

### *Giving a Quest or Task*

It is important that your slave can tell that you're setting him a submissive Quest or Task, as opposed to asking him to do something as part of daily life. Using the same wording each time can help with this. Used consistently, a phrase such as "I have a chore for you..." or "I need you to do something for me..." will become electrifying to your slave while remaining innocuous enough to be used in front of the in-laws.

You don't need to be face-to-face with your slave to issue a Quest or Task; you can also send instructions by phone or by text messaging. Sending him a text or leaving him a voice message while he's at work, informing him of a Quest he's to complete on the way home, is a sure way to brighten up his afternoon. If there's a chance that someone else might read the message (if you're using his work email address, for example) then be very sure to use innocuous wording as described above.

If you want to mix things up a bit more than a fixed formula allows, then phrase your instructions in a playfully commanding way instead. Here are three examples:

**1**

**Normal space:** "Sweetie, my phone battery hardly lasts at all any more, could you look up how to replace it and order a new one for me?"

**Mistress space:** "My phone battery is worn out so I'm giving you the task of researching and fitting a new one. I'm going to need it ready for my trip next Tuesday, so that's your deadline. Don't you dare disappoint me."

## 2

**Normal space:** "Babe, I couldn't find any red wine and I need some for the casserole for tonight, can you run out and fetch a cheap bottle?"

**Mistress space:** "I need red wine for my casserole, so you're to go and buy a bottle for me. Make sure it's appropriate for cooking. I'll be most displeased if you get the wrong kind."

## 3

**Normal space:** "I'm afraid I really yanked the front door handle earlier and it came loose again, could you have a look?"

**Mistress space:** "I ordered you to fix my front door last week, but the handle's still loose. I'm not happy about that, because I need to be sure I won't be locked out. If you know what's good for you, you won't let me down again."

Note how the "Mistress space" examples are worded so that they claim personal ownership of items (such as the front door to what is presumably a shared home) that would normally be seen as belonging to both partners. Using this kind of language reminds your slave that *you* are the one who owns things, with the obvious implication that *he* is one of the things that you own.

Also, by referring to your needs (*"I need… "*) you empower your slave to meet those needs, something he very much wishes to do; and by mentioning the consequences of failure (*"I'll be most displeased… "*, *"If you know what's good for you… "*) you remind him of his servitude to you. Afterward, his emotional payoff comes from hearing you confirm that his efforts did in fact satisfy your needs, which brings us to…

### *The Verbal Completion Bonus*

It's your slave's responsibility to complete the Quest or Task, but once he's done so you should close the Mistress-space part of the deal by checking what he did and reassuring him that you are aware that he served you, and are satisfied by the outcome he achieved.

Following on from the previous three examples:

### 1

**Normal space:** "Wow, my phone looks and works like new, thanks for taking care of that!"

**Mistress space:** "I'd have been in trouble if my phone had died, so you pleased me by meeting that tight deadline."

### 2

**Normal space:** "Thanks!" (as he brings the wine into the kitchen and hands it to her)

**Mistress space:** (playfully) "Thanks for getting that for me!" (checks the label, then raises her eyebrows at the cork) "You don't expect your Mistress to open this, do you?"

### 3

**Normal space:** "The door handle works great now, do you think it will last until we can get it replaced?"

**Mistress space:** "I'm pleased that you did such a good job of fixing my door handle. If you keep this up, *I* might keep you!"

Having given your slave the reassurance and feedback he needs, you can shift straight back into normal space. If your acknowledgement was a bit harsh, you might want to give him a smile and a "thank you" to signal that things are back to normal and that he did okay.

If you want to put a cherry on the icing for him, you could add a very minor quickie boon before you leave Mistress space. Something like a proprietary tap on the rump, just enough to let him know that his submissive service was of value to you, and you still think he's worth owning.

## *Tasks that Lead to Punishment*

If you're looking for playful reasons to punish your slave, then a completed Task offers at least three possibilities:

1. You can add a caveat to your acknowledgement and reassurance: "You cleaned that very well, but I think you missed a tiny bit there," (You brush an invisible fleck of dirt away). "Do you think you deserve to be punished for that?" The fact that you invented the dirt needs to be obvious, so that your slave understands that you are not actually unhappy with his performance, but are instead taking the opportunity to offer him a punishment boon.

2. You can give a punishment boon as a reward for a Task that he completed in an exemplary manner: "You did that so well that I want you to be able to repeat it in future, so later I'm going to fix the method in your mind with a few strokes of the whip."

3. You can give a punishment boon because your slave's completion of a Task, though successful overall, was imperfect (this does not apply if you believe the imperfection was due to your slave being lazy or trying to manipulate you): "You did a great job getting the car sparkling clean, but I see a little wax below the fender that you didn't quite buff off. You'll do better next time if I punish you for that."

## *The Bigger Picture*

I've already mentioned that the desire to "sacrifice for Mistress" is a key driver of male submission. The questing knights from the legends of King Arthur were sacrificing — sometimes their very lives — as they attempted to complete the holy quests they were given.

When your slave drives to the store, his sacrifice of time in front of the TV watching the ball game isn't exactly in the same league as those knightly quests, but the psychological principle is the same.

## Impossible Tasks

There is a place for impossible tasks in female dominant play, but the kinds of Quests and Tasks being covered here need to be doable. They can be challenging and time-consuming, there might be a risk of failure, but it should not be impossible for your slave to complete them to your satisfaction.

## Handling Failure

Occasionally, your slave is bound to get something wrong, or fail to complete a task you set. In some case he might fail spectacularly — maybe in the earlier example, while trying to replace Mistress's smartphone battery, he wrecked the phone. You wouldn't assign such a Task unless you knew your slave was competent at technical work such as repairing electronic devices, but even so, what if he messed up?

The first thing to understand is that a genuine submissive will already be beating himself up over his failure, and is probably dreading being confronted with your disappointment. Even if the task was trivial, given more as a piece of dominant play than because of a real need, he will still feel bad about failing you.

As long as your slave made a real effort, and particularly if the Task was a difficult one with an obvious risk of failure, then in most cases you'll want to cut him some slack. That doesn't mean not scolding or punishing him — punishment by Mistress is a boon, after all — but since he has only failed within your mutually-created fantasy, you should keep any scolding and punishment there (where they are actually disguised rewards, of course).

On the other hand, you are entitled to expect your slave to make his best efforts. He should complete typical domestic errands or tasks promptly and efficiently, and without unnecessarily bothering you about how he does so.

Let's imagine for a moment that he hasn't done that. Imagine that you sent him to fetch meat and potatoes and he clean forgot the meat, or came back with meat that was only a day away from its expiration date when you told him to buy fresh. If he habitually does things like that, he most likely hasn't even tried.

At this point I'm going to stop using the word "slave" to describe him, because it's not appropriate.

Such behavior, particularly if it's repeated, should make you question whether he is really interested in serving you at all; maybe he just wants the turn-on of a few kinky sessions in the bedroom. If so then that's fine; any dominant-submissive relationship has to be consensual. But if you were expecting (or have been led by him to expect) something deeper than a bit of bedroom kink, then you and he have some thinking and talking to do.

It's also possible that he's deliberately failing in order to provoke you into punishing him. In other words, he's trying to manipulate you into offering a boon. Whatever you do, don't fall for that. If this man rejects your dominance by selfishly refusing to do the tasks that you've gifted him, then you're far better off by doing them yourself, rather than by rewarding his disobedience with even more erotic attention.

If a man plays mind-games and wastes your time, instead of offering you his sincere submission, he can hardly expect your female gift of dominance in return.

### *Avoiding Micro Management*

When you command your slave to perform a Task, what you really want is for him to go away, do whatever you requested, and then return having finished it. If instead he pesters you to micro-manage things, then he's either too nervous to take responsibility for his own performance, or he's hoping to get more of your attention by conning you into taking control even of the minutest aspects of the Task.

If you'd wanted that, you'd have done it yourself...

If your slave shows these tendencies, don't indulge him. Tell him that you've made him responsible for the task, and that he needs to man up[1] and start taking that responsibility.

Of course, be sure to give your slave all the information he needs

1    Such a phrase can have a powerful motivating effect on a submissive male who is driven by the continual need to win and re-win his Mistress's approval; being seen by her as a man is fundamental to that.

to complete the task at the outset, otherwise he'll have no choice but to come back for further details. In unforeseen circumstances where he genuinely can't tell what will work best for you, it can also be reasonable for him to call you for advice.

The important attitude to cultivate is that your slave should be able to answer the following question almost instinctively: "Would Mistress benefit by being consulted on this? If not, then I need to handle it myself."

It shouldn't be that hard, given that he knows you well enough to want to be enslaved by you … and if he doesn't know you, how can he hope to serve you?

### *Slave Skills and Slave Training*

Nobody can be an expert at everything, and there are bound to be some chores that you find easier and quicker to take care of yourself. That might be because you're particular about how they're done so that nobody else could match your performance (in which case the best person for the job is already doing it), or it might just be that your slave doesn't yet have the required knack.

If that's the case, then why not instruct him to develop the knack? If "slave training" or "domestic servitude" are among his kinks, he might really appreciate this, particularly if you're prepared to be involved in guiding his program of study or playfully punishing his inevitable[1] shortcomings.

Obviously, you can't expect miracles. Nobody starts out being able to cook a delicious roast dinner or iron a blouse so it's perfectly crisp, the first time they try that skill.

If you want him to become a dab hand in the kitchen, start him out with a small number of simple recipes and put those on your meal rotation, letting him be responsible for cooking on the appropriate days. As he grows more confident, his repertoire can become larger and more ambitious. The same goes for any other chores that are unfamiliar to him but that you'd like him to share — or take over entirely.

---

1    Since you are in charge of assessing him, shortcomings really can be inevitable. A slave with a kink for strict/harsh training will, of course, *want* you to find shortcomings to punish.

Don't neglect areas where your slave is already skilled. If he's great at do-it-yourself, there's no reason why you'd have to wait for a leaky tap to be fixed, or for a shelf to be put up, ever again.

Just remember that all of the above are Tasks too, and use the forms of words, rewards and so on to help your slave understand that you are in your role of Mistress as you command him to improve or exercise his skills, and then signal your dominant appreciation of the results.

# *Reflecting on Quests and Tasks*

The questions immediately below and the space overleaf, are intended to help you gain an insight into your instinctive response to the idea of setting Quests and Tasks for your slave. The remainder of the section lets you explore your attitude to the issues surrounding any Quests and Tasks that you may choose to assign.

I am comfortable with asking my husband or boyfriend to handle chores

Yes ☐
No ☐

I am comfortable with erotically commanding my slave to do Tasks

Yes ☐
No ☐

If I erotically commanded my slave to do a Task, it would be more for his benefit than for my own

Yes ☐
No ☐

If I erotically commanded my slave to do a Task, I would feel I was unfairly exploiting his submissiveness

Yes ☐
No ☐

If I erotically commanded my slave to do a Task, any submissive enjoyment he took would be an exploitation of *me*

Yes ☐
No ☐

He should serve me without needing any rewards such as eroticized positive feedback

Yes ☐
No ☐

Rewarding my slave for valuable service would make me feel good too

Yes ☐
No ☐

Overall, my feelings about my slave's desire for servitude are:

_____

_____

_____

_____

_____

_____

_____

_____

_____

_____

_____

_____

Some areas where my slave's skills could be improved are:

_____

_____

_____

_____

_____

_____

How I think my slave would feel if he failed in a Quest or Task:

_____

_____

_____

_____

_____

_____

_____

Considering my slave's personality, the best way for me to respond to a **trivial unintended** failure would be:

_____

_____

_____

_____

_____

_____

Considering my slave's personality, the best way for me to respond to an **important unintended** failure would be:

_____

_____

_____

_____

_____

_____

If my slave failed **deliberately**, in order to manipulate me, I would:

_____

_____

_____

_____

_____

_____

Three Tasks that would benefit me but that my slave would hate:

1. _____

2. _____

3. _____

| | | |
|---|---|---|
| I'd consider giving my slave an unpleasant Task that he would hate | Yes ☐ | No ☐ |
| My slave would prefer me to do an unpleasant Task instead of assigning it to him | Yes ☐ | No ☐ |
| If I gave my slave a particularly unpleasant Task, I wouls feel obligated to reward him with a matching boon | Yes ☐ | No ☐ |

38

Some implications of my answers about unpleasant Tasks are:

_____

_____

_____

_____

_____

If my slave tried to get me to micro-manage an assigned Task, I'd:

_____

_____

_____

_____

_____

_____

# *Erotic Punishment*

"when pain is over, the remembrance of it often becomes a pleasure."

— Jane Austen —
*Persuasion*

## *Safe Words and Limits*

A safe word is an easily-remembered but seemingly irrelevant word that your slave can use if he needs you to stop or pause. Having a safe word allows your slave to beg you to stop, slow down, have mercy, and so on, without you needing to worry that he really needs you to stop or have mercy. If he did, he'd say "giraffe" — or whatever safe word you had agreed.

If you are a beginning Mistress, always agree a safe word with your slave. If he uses the safe word, you must respect it. That said, it's better not to push him to the point where he uses a safe word, since that may make you both feel bad: you for being overly harsh, and him for not being submissive enough to take the punishment you'd decided was appropriate.

As you and your slave gain experience of punishment, you may agree to forego the use of a safe word. That can ramp up the emotional intensity of what you do, by apparently removing the last vestige of control from your slave.

The reason I used the word "apparently" there is that you will still be able to observe the effect you are having on your slave; if he is trembling and weeping and begging you to stop, then as a caring Mistress you *will* stop, indeed you would have stopped long before things got to that point ... unless you'd previously agreed with him that that's where you would take him — and if you and your slave are already playing in that particular ball park, you hardly need this book.

## *Reasons for Punishment*

Punishments shouldn't be completely arbitrary, either in real life or when inflicted for erotic purposes, so do your best to offer some explanation for the punishments you inflict. The explanation should come from Mistress space, as part of your shared fantasy of dominance and submission.

It could be based around a Task or Quest that he "failed" (or that you decided to find fault with), or it might be that he neglected to observe some standing order that you have given him. It might simply be that he talked back to you in a disrespectful way.

Your own dominant desire — the fact that your slave's suffering will arouse you, or please you, or teach him to better serve you — is also a perfectly valid motivation for administering punishment. The important point is that your slave will benefit from understanding the reason he is being disciplined, whatever that may be.

Do not use erotic punishment as a response to real-world failures or shortcomings[1]. If he's done something to displease you in your daily life, you need to work through the issue not with erotic power-exchange, but by means of adult communication of a different kind.

If you are angry about some serious everyday transgression, a better way to express that would be to *withhold* the erotic attention that a punishment boon represents — not as a way of hurting him or making a move in some kind of game, but because expressing real anger through physical punishment is not healthy. There's no sense in risking hurt to your future romantic and erotic relationship by bringing that kind of psychological sickness into your bedroom. Make-up sex can be great at the end of a fight; not so much at the end of a whip.

## *Why Does He Desire Punishment?*

Of course, the answer to this question will vary from submissive male to submissive male, but certain characteristics seem to be very common:

1   Some couples aim to have a lifestyle that is female-led 24-7, so the boundary between "every day life" and "the shared fantasy of Mistress space" may be blurred or even irrelevant. However, for most readers of this book, the boundary is likely to exist and will thus be something needing respect.

- **Letting Go of Responsibility**: for a man with a high level of responsibility in every day life, surrendering means stepping away from that burden — and what better proof that he has surrendered, than that he finds himself in the role of a slave and completely unable to save himself from whatever punishment his Mistress chooses to inflict on him, no matter how painful or degrading?

- **Masochism**: the physical sensations and psychological impact of corporal punishment — of being spanked or whipped, for example — can give some men erotic pleasure, particularly when combined with other forms of sexual stimulation and activity.

- **Childhood Experience**: if a young boy is physically and/or ritualistically punished by a female carer/authority-figure for the "crime" of not pleasing her while growing up, he may subconsciously come to associate punishment and helplessness with nurture and love.

- **Feeling Valued**: when you notice, remember and punish his infractions, you show him that you think it's worth taking the time and effort to correct them; in other words, that you value him. Closely related to this is your slave's desire for your erotic attention: if you are focused on punishing him (or simply on *getting ready to punish him*) then he can feel confident that you are focused on him.

### *Anticipation*

To your slave, the erotic tension created through extended anticipation can seem just as powerful as the punishment boon itself. You can trigger that anticipation by telling him in advance — hours or days, perhaps — exactly what he has in store. Or, you can hint at your plans and leave the rest to his imagination.

If you give him some details, he gets to fully savor the anticipation of the act you have planned. If not, he gets to savor the mystery instead. By varying your approach from time to time, you keep him a little off-balance and stop the anticipatory period from feeling stale.

If you've been keeping things mysterious, the beginning of your boon is the time to reveal what he faces. A delicious way to achieve this is to have your slave, once summoned and readied for punishment, go to fetch whatever implement you mean to use. If it's a whip, cane, paddle or similar, consider allowing him to grasp or touch it only by "his end" — the striking end. The instrument's grip or handle is thus reserved for you, underlining that you are the one entitled to wield it.

Another option is to make him bring it in his mouth (again only touching "his end" of it, perhaps). To degrade him even more, you can also instruct him to go and return on all fours.

The revelation of what you will use on your slave doesn't end his sense of anticipation, instead it kicks it into overdrive: his brain will now get to work on imagining in exquisite detail how the instrument will feel. Also, he still doesn't know when the business will begin, how severe it will be, how long it will continue — or what intermissions and other entertainments you might have planned.

So, have him prepared and positioned for whatever you have in mind, and then just pause. Allow him the leisure to tremble and be afraid. If you like, tease him by stroking him with your hands or with the instrument, or by musing on whether you've changed your mind about the kind of punishment to administer. Perhaps ask him if he deserves to be punished at all …

(Of course he deserves to be punished; teasing has its place but you don't want to bring this man you care for all this way, only to short-circuit him now).

Once you do begin to administer the punishment, there's still no rush. Vary the pacing of your whip strokes (or whatever other kind of sensation you are inflicting) — don't pause for so long as to risk boredom for either of you, but do allow some time for him to obsess about what comes next. Is that swishing sound you cutting the air, or aiming another stroke at his buttocks? Are you just resting your whip hand for a while, or is his ordeal over, or will you move on to some other kind of erotic torment?

Do take into account the severity of your strokes when deciding on pacing. He will need more recovery time if you are striking hard with a cane or a riding crop, than if you are striking more gently or using a punishment device that is really more of a toy.

You can also create tension by mixing things up. For example: deliver a flurry of gentler blows (directed to the same spot, these will still build up to significant pain), then give him a rest, then strike harder, then repeat.

In this way, you create unpredictable (to him) intervals during which the self-tormenting power of his own mind goes to work, greatly amplifying your physical torments and reducing the level of actual punishment required to get him to the level of submissive or masochistic fulfillment that he desires.

### *Setting the Scene*

The most natural place for a punishment boon is the bedroom. It is your most private and intimate space; it is usually easy to control the lighting and mood; it has the advantage of being equipped with a bed which (as well as its obvious vanilla-sex uses) may serve as a platform where your slave can be arranged and presented, perhaps even tied down, ready for punishment.

One way to begin is to withdraw to your bedroom to prepare, leaving your slave with instructions to present himself there in exactly fifteen minutes' time, freshly showered, shaved and naked. If you go to that level of detail, use a timer to ensure that he's punctual. A routine like this, used consistently and repeatedly, will soon develop into a powerful erotic ritual as described in the chapter *Ritual and Role-Play* on page 63.

Despite the fact that your slave will be undressed while you will be wearing whatever you choose, ensure that the room is at a temperature that suits you. Your slave's chilliness doesn't matter within reason; he is here to suffer and serve, not to be made overly comfortable.

Dim the lights, or turn them out entirely and use candles instead. If you like, have some appropriate music playing. All such preparations should either be done by you personally before the punishment boon commences, or performed by your slave under your close supervision as part of the boon. Take the opportunity to correct and rebuke any minor errors he makes in following your instructions; keeping maximum personal control over every detail of the setting reinforces the idea that this is your personal domain and that your word here is law.

The slave's mental state will be impacted by the choice of space. As I mentioned, your bedroom has several qualities that make it a suitable location, but what if you wish to push your slave outside that comfort zone? A part of your home that feels less like a sanctuary, somewhere that does not carry the same connotation of privacy, will put him in a completely different head space. Moving the punishment out of a bedroom and onto an adjacent upstairs landing, for example, can make a psychological difference to your slave that's out of all proportion to the distance involved.

Another piece of scene-setting to consider, is whether to place your slave in bondage during the punishment boon — whether as a separate part of the boon, or to secure him while you administer the punishment itself. If he's already dressed in "slave accoutrements" such as a leather collar and wrist cuffs, then it's both easy and natural to secure him (send him ahead of time on a Quest to the hardware store if necessary, to get any chains, shackles or padlocks that you might need).

The experience of being in bondage will heighten his feeling of vulnerability, while the familiar, snug sensation of ropes or straps can also be a comfort to your slave. The more secure the bondage, the more mental impact it will have. Tight but gentle rope bondage might feel good to him, but it will probably not bring the same feeling of instant helplessness as that achieved by the clicking sound of a pair of handcuffs closing about his wrists as you secure him to the headboard of your bed.

**Safety First!**

*Never leave your slave alone while he's secured in bondage, and never place anything around his neck that could cut off his breathing. Always have a way (such as a safe word) for him to signal that he needs to be released. If he's gagged or otherwise unable to speak, ensure that you have a pre-agreed, non-verbal signal he can use if needed. If using anything that locks, keep a spare key close at hand.*

*For maximum safety when chaining/padlocking him to any immovable object, use securing points made with nylon rope or plastic cable ties. This arrangement can be made completely escape-proof as far as your slave is concerned, but as long as you keep a cutting tool handy, you will always be able to release him even if a lock jams.*

## Instruments

The best instrument to use as a beginning Mistress is your palm. Spanking is less intimidating (both to you and your slave) than actual punishment toys. As the slave feels sensation, so do you; his buttocks (being much more sensitive) will sting more than your hand, but your hand *will* begin to sting if you continue for long. This is useful feedback that can help you build confidence about what you are doing.

There's a quality of intimacy to a formal, over-the-knee bare-bottomed spanking, something that sets it apart from what can be achieved with a paddle or a whip. It stems partly from the physical closeness involved, but I believe that much of it comes from the fact that an over-the-knee spanking is typically seen, in our culture, as a punishment for children. By using it on your slave you are implicitly assigning him a more junior status, and casting yourself in the role of the person who cares for him, makes decisions on his behalf, and when necessary, administers a loving correction.

If you wish to administer harsher punishments, or if you want something that *seems* more cruel, or even if you just wish to spare the stinging of your palm, then you'll want to consider a different instrument. You might begin by looking around your home: something like a wooden spatula from the kitchen can serve perfectly well. When you're ready, consider acquiring one of the many specialized punishment toys that are available:

- A light flogger with soft tails is a good beginner's choice. Despite seeming fearsome (its design resembles that of the "cat-o'nine tails" used historically in organizations such as the British Navy to inflict very severe punishments) it causes surprisingly little pain. Don't worry if your slave is disappointed by this; your right and need to proceed at your own pace, outweigh his desire for intense sensation.

- The tawse is a short, stiffened leather strap that has the benefit of being highly controllable; its length and stiffness tend to make it go where you want it to, while the relatively large contact area (particularly with a plain tawse as opposed to a split-ended one) means it won't cut or leave sharp welts. In former times, the tawse was used on the palms of disobedient children in some British and Irish schools. You can use it in the same way on your slave, but it comes into its own when applied to his behind.

- Paddles are also controllable. They tend to deliver a deep, thudding sensation; if you're looking for a more stinging effect then try a lighter and more flexible paddle — although in that case, I would personally bypass this choice and go for a tawse instead.

- The cane has connotations of school punishment that are even stronger than those of the tawse. This instrument is fierce and you should leave its use until you are comfortable and confident with the more controllable alternatives.

- Finally, the riding crop is the instrument with the most fetish symbolism. As a beginner, you should look for an example with a generous soft leather tongue; you can create a satisfying snap on his skin by flicking with this, without causing much pain. If you wish to apply a stronger treatment, use the shaft of the crop rather than the tongue — but as with the cane, it takes practice before you can do this controllably.

Speaking of practice: before using a new instrument on your slave, you should work with it for a while in order to gain confidence with it. Try it on the sofa cushions or bedspread to learn how it handles, and how to place strokes accurately. Flick it (using the power of your wrist only) against your palm, lightly at first and then more forcefully, to get an idea of how the intensity changes. Also experiment by stroking or caressing your own skin with various parts of the instrument, to gain some understanding of the sensations you will be giving to your slave when you do the same to him.

### *Administering Punishment*

It's worth re-stating the importance of pace: vary the tempo to create anticipation, and also to take account of your slave's responses. This applies even before the punishment proper has started, since you can use this period to prepare your slave physically and mentally, by attending to the part of his body that is to be punished.

This could be as simple as caressing the skin with your hand, your whip, or anything else that will cause intense erotic sensation. You could apply oil or lotion, both as a gesture of preparation and to intensify the coming sensations. You could arrange him with his legs spread sufficiently for you to caress his penis and scrotum, or to very gently apply the tip of your whip.

The most satisfactory part of his body to spank or whip is the "sweet spot" near the base of his buttocks, where he has the maximum padding. As you move up from the sweet spot, the amount of padding diminishes, so strokes placed here will hurt more. Avoid striking toward top of his butt where there is little padding between the skin and the bone, because this will cause serious pain and possible damage. Every man is a little different, so take the time to explore his anatomy with your hands so that you have a sense of how he carries his padding of muscle and fat, where it is thick, and where it thins out.

The intensity of punishment is also affected by his posture. Bending him over stretches the skin tautly and makes the punishment harsher, while unbending him loosens it, allowing more "bounce" to absorb the energy of your strokes (and if you enjoy seeing his flesh jiggle as your blows land, to delight your eyes).

Curling into a ball is an instinctive protective response, so ordering him to do the opposite of this, and to arch his back, will also make him feel more vulnerable.

Light taps, even with a fierce implement like the shaft of a crop, can be repeated swiftly; you might wish to view a flurry of blows as a single stroke and then play with the timing between flurries. Heavier strokes need to be spread out so he has time to recover.

Allow more time, too, as the punishment proceeds and begins to take its toll on your slave's ability to withstand it. Early on, if he's shrugging off your punishment or scornfully asking when you plan to start, you can strike harder and more quickly. Once your slave's resistance begins to break down, you can slow the pace.

Listen to the changing sounds he makes and observe his body language. Stoic grunts may change into pained gasps or yelps; an obediently arched back and pertly presented rump might hunch protectively in response to a fierce stroke. These are signs that the punishment is beginning to get to him. Depending on your preference and his needs, you may wish to stop, or to push him further, or perhaps to pause to comfort him (a loving, sympathetic kiss should perk him up considerably, as should the healing sensation of your cool caressing palms — or perhaps a drizzle of soothing lotion — upon his burning rump. It is also possible to take a break and have him serve you in some other way, before resuming his punishment once he has had time to recover.

Be aware that lotion might comfort him, but its moisturizing properties can make him feel any further whip strokes even more keenly.

Warming balms (the kind often used to relieve joint aches or nasal congestion) containing menthol, camphor, mint or other fiery ingredients will also amplify the sensations you create, and can thus serve to spice up a punishment even more.

## *What to Do Next?*

It's natural to reach a point in a punishment boon where you find yourself needing a moment to decide what to do next — or even wondering, *"What does he really want me to do next?"*

If so, it will help if you understand the most important thing that's going on in your slave's head during a punishment boon:

**What he really wants is for you to continue to be in control**

So, if you need some time to plan your next move, use the control that you have — that he *needs* you to have — to create a breathing space. It can be as simple as ordering him to kneel or to stand in a particular way until told otherwise, or to walk around the room for you ... with his hands on his head, if you like; something that would seem silly or embarrassing in real life, will feel natural during a punishment boon, and the more detailed your instructions, the more he has to focus on as he strives to comply with them to your satisfaction.

What is really significant to your slave is not the detail of what he is required to do, but the fact that you have required him to do it — and that his performance is subject to your scrutiny and judgement.

If you prefer, have him do something to please you more directly. Moving away from some simple command, and instead allowing him the opportunity to perform some more intimate service for you, lets him show his mettle more directly and holds a greater sense of risk and reward for him.

Either way, hearing and obeying your commands, and later receiving your feedback, reward and/or punishment, will bring your slave the satisfaction of being subject to your female authority and judgement. And, the more ways you can work in to *please yourself while apparently being cruel to him*, the happier your slave will be.

## *Alternative Punishments*

Besides the spankings and paddlings described up to now, there are other ways of causing physical pain or discomfort to your slave.

Here are some examples of "non-corporal" forms of punishment that are nevertheless physical in nature:

- Ordering him to maintain a stress position, for example kneeling on a hard wooden floor or a bristled mat; or standing with arms outstretched while gripping light weights (chosen to cause difficulty and discomfort while enabling him to support them for long enough to make the punishment meaningful).

- Applying nipple clamps. You can substitute clothes pins, but ensure the tension is suitable and modify them as necessary — have your slave research and perform this as a Task, if you like.

- Subjecting him to cold- or heat-play with ice cubes or droplets of candle wax.

- Ordering him to perform exercises such as push ups, squats, or weights; or to work until he has burned a certain number of calories on an exercise bicycle; or to serve as your "galley slave" on a rowing machine.

- Ordering him to get under a cold shower for a brief period; it doesn't take long to get the point across!

- Blindfolding him during any other punishment to heighten the sensations and the feeling of vulnerability.

Not every form of punishment is suitable for every slave. For example, if your slave has problems with his knee joints, you won't want to force him into a kneeling stress position; if he has cardiovascular problems, you won't want to push him into intense exercise activities beyond those recommended by his physician.

On the other hand, if he's in good health and lazy about exercising, this kind of punishment or improvement program could benefit his fitness level and physique in ways that go beyond the submissive/erotic.

## *Reluctance and Rebellion*

Your slave may welcome and enjoy certain punishments, even ones that are painful and/or humiliating. Those will be the punishments that push his submissive buttons, thus rewarding him for the pain he endures (the pain is inextricably linked to the reward).

Most often, these punishments will be the ones that carry erotic symbolism with them — the fact that a punishment is personally administered by you, his Mistress, being an important part of that symbolism.

Other punishments may be less welcome, particularly at the time they are given. A particularly harsh whipping, one that goes from being erotic to being punitive (you can tell the difference by checking if he has a hard-on; as long as he does, the experience remains erotic for him) might fall into this category for some slaves. So might being made to stand under a cold shower.

In these cases, your slave might show strong reluctance to comply with his punishment. He might beg, wheedle, plead, or try to negotiate. You may need to flick him with a riding crop to demonstrate that you mean business. As long as he does not use his safe-word, you shouldn't feel guilty about pressing on — he *wants* to be pushed into accepting your punishment.

If you're not using a safe-word, then you and he have already agreed that his fate is to be in your hands, and you should know him well enough to be aware if you are pushing him into a mental place where he should not be made to go. If you're not both fully comfortable with that level of responsibility and intimacy, don't play without a safe word.

A truly submissive slave will not actually rebel against you; even if there's a show of reluctance he will eventually accept his punishment and will comply with commands that you give as part of this: to strip, to fetch the whip, to assume the required position, or to be bound if that's what you wish for him.

That said, a certain level of "pretend" rebellion can be fun, as long as it is clear that his resistance exists only at your sufferance. The next chapter (*Ritual and Role-Play*) covers several scenarios that involve a portrayal of resistance, but this kind of rebelliousness is, of course, just a different level of compliance with your wishes, since it is you who sets the limits of the role-play. The appearance of defiance (and the breaking-down of that defiance through your feminine power) is something both you and your slave can enjoy.

If you encounter a serious rebellion that goes beyond role-play — if he refuses to accept your whip, for example, or if he uses superior physical strength to prevent you doing as you wish with him — the bottom line is that you are not obliged to try to overcome him. If he resists in a way that's not fun for you and that plainly is not an invitation for you to "overpower" him, then make it clear that he has one last chance to obey you. If he still resists, tell him that you're happy he's been cured of his previous submissive tendencies, and that he can now put his clothes back on and continue with his day, as you will continue with yours.

If you get to this point, *do not back down*. You have declared your boon to be over. Re-starting it because of his promises or wheedling, would be putting him in control.

Later, you'll need talk about what went wrong. If there was some issue that can be talked out and solved, then fine. If you mutually agree that your dominance-submission games need less intensity, that's fine too. However, it's also possible that you won't be able to have this kind of relationship with this man, despite what he thinks he wants. It's entirely up to you whether you give him a second chance, and if so how long he must wait and what he must do to earn it.

## *Aftercare*

Even moderately intense dominance play can leave your slave bruised, exhausted, trippy, perhaps even shaking as if from cold. He might need to re-hydrate with water or a sports drink, and to boost his energy with a chocolate bar. He might have feelings of inadequacy and even guilt, convincing himself that the boon you provided was done to please him, and that you didn't really enjoy it. He might feel embarrassed and ashamed about what he has allowed — *needed* — you to do.

You, too, might feel exhausted. You might see the welts you've left on his skin and be worried that you've overdone things, so that you need his reassurance that you didn't stray too far from pleasure and into pain. Maybe you just need to know that despite treating him cruelly, you still have your slave's love and submission.

It is impossible for any of us to predict what aftercare someone else might need. Some slaves feel the effects of an intense punishment boon for days; others just carry on as if not much has happened. Some slaves can end up feeling depressed, particularly if intense verbal humiliation has been used on them.

The main thing is to be aware that you and your slave should take whatever time is needed to gradually return to normal and to reassure and comfort one another so that neither feels abandoned. Cuddling can help; so can hot chocolate. For a couple in a caring relationship, the most essential aftercare medicine is the mutual knowledge and love that goes with that; as long as you and your slave have those, the rest will follow.

# *Reflecting on Erotic Punishment*

The purpose of this section is to help you explore and clarify your feelings about physically punishing your slave. Particularly if you are an inexperienced Mistress, you might find that you are not yet ready to address some of these questions. If so, you are of course free to leave them blank for now.

I will communicate a safe word to my slave for use     Yes ☐
during any punishment I inflict on him     No ☐

If using a safe word, it is:

_____

The idea of punishing my slave...[1]     Arouses Me ☐
    Disturbs Me ☐
    Intrigues Me ☐

The idea that my slave might wish me to     Arouses Me ☐
punish him...     Disturbs Me ☐
    Intrigues Me ☐

A punishment can sometimes also be a reward     Yes ☐
    No ☐

I think my slave would like more severe punishment     Yes ☐
than I would be prepared to give     No ☐

I think I would like to give more severe punishment     Yes ☐
than my slave would be able to tolerate     No ☐

[1] A single idea can be arousing, intriguing and disturbing at the same time, so check multiple boxes if appropriate.

The ordeal I think my slave would fear most (or desire least) is:

_____

_____

_____

_____

_____

_____

because _____

_____

_____

_____

_____

_____

_____

56

The ordeal I think my slave would fear least (or desire most) is:

_____

_____

_____

_____

_____

_____

because _____

_____

_____

_____

_____

_____

_____

Overall, my feelings about punishing my slave are:

_____

_____

_____

_____

_____

_____

_____

_____

_____

_____

_____

_____

I would punish my slave for my own pleasure · · · · · · Yes ☐ / No ☐

I would punish my slave to improve his behavior · · · · · · Yes ☐ / No ☐

I would punish my slave for "made-up" reasons within our shared fantasy · · · · · · Yes ☐ / No ☐

I would punish my slave to secretly reward him · · · · · · Yes ☐ / No ☐

I believe that my slave could gain pleasure later from a punishment he was reluctant to accept at the time · · · · · · Yes ☐ / No ☐

Three possible reasons for punishing my slave:

1. _____

2. _____

3. _____

Three punishments I could inflict on my slave without striking him:

1. _____

2. _____

3. _____

I think my slave *desires* to be punished...                    Yes ☐
                                                                 No ☐

because _____

_____

_____

_____

_____

Some implications of my previous two answers are:

_____

_____

_____

_____

_____

_____

I think my slave *deserves* to be punished...   Yes ☐
                                                 No ☐

because _____

_____

_____

_____

_____

Some implications of my previous two answers are:

_____

_____

_____

_____

_____

_____

Some reassurances I might need after punishing my slave are:

_____

_____

_____

_____

_____

Some reassurances my slave might need after I have punished him are:

_____

_____

_____

_____

_____

_____

I am mentally and emotionally resilient                Yes ☐
                                                       No ☐

I believe my slave is mentally and emotionally resilient   Yes ☐
                                                       No ☐

I plan to engage in particularly demanding             Yes ☐
dominance games with my slave                          No ☐


With the above three answers in mind, my feelings about aftercare are:

_____

_____

_____

_____

_____

_____

_____

# Ritual and Role-Play

"Being your slave, what should I do but tend
Upon the hours and times of your desire?
I have no precious time at all to spend,
Nor services to do, till you require."

— William Shakespeare —
*Sonnet 57*

## Rituals

Traditionally, a ritual is a sequence of (often religious) behavior that is observed according to a particular form. In its erotic sense, the word signifies a sequence of acts that is repeated until it becomes comfortably familiar, taking on a symbolic significance to the lovers who follow it. So, the ritual parts of your domination over your slave are those that you and he perform repeatedly in the same way. Just as religious rituals confirm that their celebrants and congregations share the same faith and form of worship, so do erotic rituals bind couples who follow them more closely as Mistress and slave.

If you have a particular way of touching him to signify that you are giving him a Task or Quest, that's a ritual. Similarly, if he must always present himself naked for punishment, or if you always send him to fetch the whip, then his nakedness and the humiliating task of fetching the instrument of his own punishment, become a ritualized part of the punishment boon.

Unlike many religious rituals, erotic rituals should generally be kept simple so that they can flow with little conscious effort. Through familiarity, erotic ritual becomes comforting and peaceful, even if it is part of something exciting. The ritual's fixed form eliminates anxiety as the participant's minds are freed from having to think about what they should do next.

Repeating the same ritual over and over again within a highly erotic context, charges the ritual itself with eroticism, to the point where you and/or your slave begin to miss the ritual if you have to skip it for some reason.

## *Creating and Establishing Rituals*

There is no point in creating rituals that don't have deep meaning for one or the other or both of you, so the best place to look for ideas is in the boons and other interactions you play out together. If you liked some symbolic act that you commanded or that he volunteered, it's a candidate to be made into a ritual. When you ask your slave what really worked for him, his answers may give you other suitable ideas.

Here are some possibilities to consider, ranging from ritualized tasks in which he serves you each time in the same way, to rituals of discipline that could become a routine part of every punishment boon or reserved for when you wish to make a particularly strong impression:

- Have him bring you a cup of your preferred drink each morning, and then present it in a specific way.

- Have him perform some regular task each week (such as polishing your shoes, ironing your clothes, cleaning the bathroom) and then inspect his work with him.

- Have him always open and hold the door for you.

- Have a ritualized[1] way of letting him know when he is to give you cunnilingus.

- Have a ritualized way for him to ask to give you cunnilingus.

- Keep a special candle that is only lit during punishment boons and extinguished when they end. If you wish, make your slave responsible for lighting and extinguishing the candle.

- Place a collar on him in a particular way, for example having him bring you the collar and then kneel before you while you fasten it around his neck.

- Make him ritually ask to have his bad behavior corrected through punishment; make him thank you afterwards.

---

1    Ritualized in the sense of using the same specific command or signal every time.

- Make him kiss the instrument of punishment before and/or after the punishment itself.

- Have him remove or trim his body hair, particularly his pubic hair[1], and ritually inspect him at intervals to ensure he has done so efficiently.

- Send him to stand in the corner for a period.

- Make him write an apology, or "lines" as in the old school punishment where a misbehaving pupil would be required to neatly write out a line suited to their crime, such as "I must not talk in class," a given number of times.

The ritual nature of any punishment depends on continuity. If he is punished with "corner time", you can turn it into a ritual by making it the same corner every time, and using the same words to command it and to signify when it's over. For a written punishment, you can turn it into a ritual by having him sit in the same place, dressed (or undressed) in the same way, and with pen and paper that are reserved for this purpose. These rituals eroticize the punishment for him, meaning he will be aroused by the ordeal. If you ever need to punish your slave more seriously, consider removing any ritual elements to make your displeasure clear to him.

In case there's any doubt: rituals are not just for him. If you'd like to start the day with a cuddle followed by him preparing breakfast, that can be part of your and his morning ritual. If you need an extended shoulder rub each evening — for however long it takes to ease away the knots left by a stressful day — make that a ritual too.

To establish a ritual you and your slave must follow it consistently. Rituals that seem silly or embarrassing at first, can develop into powerful symbolic expressions of dominance, submission and eroticism — but only if you both keep them up.

1 Removal of pubic hair is a common symbol of submission. The possession of pubic hair signifies full adulthood, while its removal symbolizes reduced status and demonstrates that the submissive male (and particularly the part of him thus exposed) is your property.

## Rituals of Degradation

The erotic rituals of dominance and submission almost invariably involve some degree of degradation or humiliation; these qualities are a large part of what gives the rituals their power. At first, the idea of being "ritually degraded" can sound like a negative, undesirable thing, but to your slave it is probably the opposite, since the need to feel erotically degraded can be an essential part of a submissive male's make-up.

Here is a dictionary definition of the word, "Degrade":

1. To reduce from a higher to a lower rank or degree; to lower in rank to deprive of office or dignity; to strip of honors; as, to degrade a nobleman, or a general officer.

2. To reduce in estimation, character, or reputation; to lessen the value of; to lower the physical, moral, or intellectual character of; to debase; to bring shame or contempt upon; to disgrace; as, vice degrades a man.

Reduction in rank and loss of dignity is an inevitable part of the role that your slave has taken on; degradation goes with the territory. There is no way to play dominance-submission games without the slave being assigned a lower rank than the Mistress, and thus being "degraded".

In short: by degrading your slave, you are also fulfilling him.

## Degradation vs Humiliation

Degradation and Humiliation seem almost like interchangeable words, but there is an important nuance of difference between them.

Compare the following dictionary definition of the word, "Humiliate" with the previous definition of "Degrade":

"Humiliate: To reduce to a lower position in one's own eyes, or in the eyes of others; to humble; to mortify."

Notice that crucial difference: "in one's own eyes."

- Degrading your slave is about stripping away his usual status and confirming your role as his Mistress. It normally involves things happening to his body. If you remove his right to wear clothes, or force him to be collared, or send him away to fetch the whip with which he is to be punished, these are all physical actions that demonstrate his enslavement.

- Humiliating your slave is about stripping away his sense of self-worth. It normally involves belittling statements intended to affect his mind. If you tell him (particularly when he is in a vulnerable state due to being deep in submission) that he is useless, lazy, unattractive, unlovable or pathetic, then you are not just giving him fulfillment by reducing him to a lower symbolic status, you may also be undermining his sense of self-worth.

Both degradation and humiliation can be highly arousing for a submissive person, though not all slaves enjoy humiliation. As we've seen, reduction in status is a fundamental aspect of dominance-submission play, but humiliation is an optional element — and it's one you must approach with great caution, even if your slave is really turned on by the experience of you belittling him in this way.

The fact that humiliation is an attack on self-worth is exactly why some slaves crave it; self-worth is the foundation of personal power, so stripping it away helps satisfy the slave's need to become utterly powerless. The problem is that undermining his sense of self-worth can be damaging later. The notion that he has a tiny penis that could never satisfy any woman might seem hot to him when he's deep into a punishment boon, but the memory might mortify him as he dwells on your words the next day.

As a caring Mistress you can avoid this risk by not using strong humiliation; at the very least you must be familiar enough with your slave's mental state to avoid any "hot issues" arising from his childhood or other past circumstances. If you do use strong humiliation, don't neglect the appropriate mutual aftercare during which you can gently reassure him that he's okay, while he reassures you that you haven't gone too far.

## *Role-Play*

You are automatically role-playing each time you give a boon: you take on the character of "cruel Mistress"; he takes on the character of "submissive slave"; together you create a shared fantasy around these roles.

If you wish to explore a deeper kind of role-playing, you can experiment with personas and stories that are more fully-formed than the basic "Mistress" and "slave" models, but that are still chosen to maintain the dynamic of dominance, submission and erotic torment. How about:

- The Pirate Queen and her helpless hostage; perhaps the Pirate Queen suspects that the hostage knows the whereabouts of a long-lost treasure map?

- The Roman noblewoman and the new slave she's assessing; if he's not satisfactory he risks being sold off to work in the salt mines instead of as her bed slave...

- The Stern Headmistress and the lazy student; she is eager to get to the bottom of why his grades have been slipping...

- The well-armed Householder and the bungling burglar; he will end up paying a delightful price for his intrusion...

- The Inquisitrix and the Goddess-denying heretic strapped to her rack (that in a certain light looks suspiciously like her bed)...

- The musket-toting Southern Belle and the captured Union soldier in possession of vital military plans...

- The Sorceress and the demon trapped in her pentagram; maybe if she can magically force him into chains with her riding crop (I mean, her wand!), she can safely allow him out of the circle and into her bed...

A role-playing scenario can be as simple or as elaborate as you like. At its most ambitious, it's a small dramatic production of your own, so if you've ever imagined yourself in a role that can be played out erotically, this is your chance. There is naturally some preparation work for you to do (assisted by your slave, who probably needs to know what's planned in any case). You'll sketch out what is to happen, and maybe acquire or create costumes and props if that side of the fantasy appeals to you.

Brief your slave ahead of time if you wish to "direct" his performance. If he's the lazy student who's failed an important test, do you want him to be insolent and full of himself until you bring him to heel, or do you prefer to have him timid and worried about being expelled? Is there a hidden reason for his poor grades, one that you can force out of him (maybe even one that he could make up himself)? If he's a captive soldier, do you want him to be defiant, blustering, defeated, injured in the recent battle?

You may like to add props to explain why he must obey you and submit to whatever torment you have in mind for him. A Southern Belle probably could not coerce a northern soldier, unless she was armed; the same goes for a Householder and a burglar. You can use toys as props, or pre-agree which safe item will stand in as the threatening object.

The need to plan things in advance applies doubly if your slave is supposed to know a vital plot detail such as a secret. You can use these secrets — and their inevitable discovery — by having your slave write the "secret" and hide it somewhere in the room you plan to use. Then you'll try to make him give up the secret using whatever means you choose. If your slave holds out long enough to impress you (set a timer, if you like) maybe he'll get a bonus of your choosing before the end of the boon...

As always, role-playing is at your discretion. It takes confidence to enter and act out a fantasy role, particularly as there is going to be a certain amount of "making it up as you go along". Only proceed if you actively wish to do so. If you do, remember that planning out plot details like secrets, goals and hidden agendas gives you and your slave something to hang your "performances" on, and makes it easier for you both to relax and have fun rather than fixating on what to say and do.

## *Online Role-Play*

If taking on the persona of Mistress in your bedroom is quite enough live role-playing for you at the moment, then playing on-line can offer a less stressful avenue to explore.

The advantage of playing on-line instead of live in your bedroom, is that you can experience whatever scenario you like without the pressure of props, costumes, or thinking up dialog on the spur of the moment. You and your slave may then find it easier to express yourselves, to use evocative language without embarrassment, even to say things you might otherwise feel unable to express.

You can both take (and invent) things at your own pace while enjoying the luxury of having the story unfold in your imaginations, instead of being limited to what is possible in the real world. If you like, you can have castles and flying carpets and dragons…

If you do take this route and find you enjoy it, then there's nothing stopping you from adding in some live role-play sessions later, when you feel ready.

Online role-playing is a widespread activity, with web forums existing both for erotic and non-erotic variations. Of course, there's no requirement to join or use a forum for online role-play with your partner; a pair of email accounts or even a couple of smart phones, plus two human imaginations, is all you need. Searching out an online forum that you like can still be worthwhile though, even if it's just as a source for ideas.

# *Reflecting on Ritual and Role-Play*

This section is for you to consider and explore the kinds of erotic or other rituals and role-play that you might enjoy with your slave.

I view rituals of dominance and submission as[1]

Arousing ☐

Embarrassing ☐

Intriguing ☐

A way to control my slave's mental state ☐

A way to direct my own mental state ☐

It would be easy to find rituals that would please both myself and my slave…

Yes ☐

No ☐

…because _____

_____

_____

_____

_____

_____

_____

---

1   As usual, check multiple boxes if appropriate.

Three explicitly erotic rituals that might please or serve me:

1. _____

2. _____

3. _____

Three rituals (not directly erotic) that might please or serve me:

1. _____

2. _____

3. _____

Three explicitly erotic rituals I think would please my slave:

1. _____

2. _____

3. _____

Three rituals (not directly erotic) that I think would please my slave:

1. _____

2. _____

3. _____

Three role-play scenarios that would mainly be for me[1]:

1. _____

2. _____

3. _____

Three role-play scenarios that would mainly be for my slave:

1. _____

2. _____

3. _____

---

1 Feel free to choose scenarios that do not involve eroticism or power-exchange, if you so desire.

Three role-play scenarios that would be for both of us:

1. _____

2. _____

3. _____

| | |
|---|---|
| I would feel uncomfortable or embarrassed about taking part in a detailed role-play scenario | Yes ☐ No ☐ |
| As a girl, I used to enjoy "pretend" games | Yes ☐ No ☐ |
| As a woman, I have enjoyed masked balls, fancy dress, murder-mystery parties or similar | Yes ☐ No ☐ |

The level of planning and preparation I would put in to a scenario

A detailed plan by me ☐
A detailed plan by my slave ☐
A detailed plan, done together ☐
A brief outline will suffice ☐
Choose an idea and wing it ☐

I would get scenario ideas from

My own imagination ☐
Suggestions by my slave ☐
My favorite movies, books or plays ☐
Current or historical events ☐
Browsing the internet ☐

I would feel more comfortable about playing out
a scenario on-line than in-the-flesh

Yes ☐
No ☐

On-line role-play could offer a way to ease
the challenges of a long-distance relationship

Yes ☐
No ☐

My taboo subjects (if any) that should *not* be explored in role-play:

_____

_____

_____

_____

_____

My taboo subjects (if any) that *could* be beneficially explored:

_____

_____

_____

_____

_____

A role-playing fantasy that intrigues me is:

_____

_____

_____

_____

_____

_____

_____

_____

_____

_____

_____

_____

# *Orgasm Control*

"Virtue is the fount whence honour springs."

— Christopher Marlowe —
*Tamburlaine the Great*

Left to his own devices, the typical male (whether submissive or not) will regularly masturbate to the point of ejaculation in order to release erotic tension. Even if he's regularly receiving the ministrations of a loving partner who sees to his satisfaction in every way she can, he may still masturbate "just because" … it's something he learned to do in his teens, he probably did it compulsively (and perfectly healthily) through that part of his life, and even as a grown man he finds that it remains a habit that he enjoys.

There are several reasons why this can be undesirable in a female-led relationship:

- Frequent ejaculation satisfies his sex drive, so that the energy that comes from his libido — the erotic and romantic attention could be spent on you, to his benefit as well as to yours — ends up spent in his hand.

- While masturbating, a submissive man is going to imagine fantasy scenarios of dominance and submission that work for him as perfectly as possible. There's nothing wrong with a man enjoying a good sexual fantasy, as long as it doesn't negatively influence his expectations and needs outside of that fantasy. Earlier in this book, I cautioned you to be on guard for men fixated on an idealized vision of their leather-clad, stiletto-heeled Dominatrix, a fantasy creation that no real-life partner could possibly match. Well, if they didn't meet these women in real life, how did they burden themselves with such an impossible aspiration? I'll give you one guess.

- None of the above is compatible with your slave's submissive desire to serve you and sacrifice for you. Succumbing to the instant gratification of an orgasm, can get in the way of a long-term fulfillment that would meet his submissive needs far more effectively.

⚢

Perhaps the most complete and intimate act of surrender that a male slave can offer his Mistress, is to give her control over when and how he receives sexual stimulation, and most particularly over when and how he is permitted to ejaculate. The more complete this control, the more perfectly submissive he can feel.

By the same token, one of the most intimate and erotic statements of ownership that a dominant female can make, is to lovingly and teasingly exercise that control.

As well as the symbolic "Mistress-slave" implication that you own his genitals along with the pleasurable acts and sensations he associates with them, there are several other benefits:

- It is natural to wish to please someone who can offer or withhold a deeply-desired reward. After a period of chastity, the gift of sexual stimulation and possible ejaculation, will be at the very top of his list of "desired rewards" — and you are the one person in the wide world who can grant that reward, or withhold it. If there's anything that can make a submissive male more happily and consistently attentive to his Mistress, I have yet to discover it.

- This expression of your ownership will satisfy his submissive needs in a unique way, because the full power of his male libido will be working in the same direction as your own female authority. His "vanilla" need for sex will join his "kinky" need for submission, in driving him to obey and please you.

- It opens up new ways to punish him. As well as a punishment taking the form of an action (such as a whipping) it can also take the form of an *in*action (such as being left frustrated for another day or another week).

- It brings the possibility of introducing new and erotically-charged toys in the form of chastity belts or lockable tubes, if you wish to go in this direction.

## *Two Kinds of Male Chastity*

The first way in which your slave can remain chaste for you could not be simpler: he refrains from masturbating. If he has the submissive self-discipline to manage it, this "honor-based chastity" is by far the less troublesome way for him to surrender control over his orgasms, and for both of you to enjoy the corresponding benefits.

The second way is for you to enforce his chastity by securing his penis in a specially-made lockable device, with you becoming his "keyholder". Male chastity devices are generally designed to prevent the wearer from having an erection (or in many cases, to allow partial erections that are more frustrating than fulfilling). Once locked in, his opportunities for sexual pleasure or even for normal arousal, will become extremely constrained.

Device-based chastity is much more complicated and demanding (for you as well as for him) than the honor-based alternative, but it does offer some powerful erotic compensations. As soon as you snap that lock into place and put the key away, his submission goes from being voluntary to being compelled — having placed himself so completely at your mercy, he will have the feeling that it is *physically necessary* for him to please you — and to avoid incurring your displeasure. On your side, you have the knowledge that he is under your control to a degree that you might never have imagined possible.

Still, if you and he are beginners, and if he is sufficiently strong-willed in his obedience to be able to refrain from masturbation at your command, then there's a lot to be said for starting with honor-based chastity. For one thing, you and he already have all the equipment you need! Also, you won't need to deal with the demands and complexities of device-based chastity, including possible disappointments about devices that are not completely secure, or that chafe him excessively.

A middle way is to purchase a device as a toy, and to use it for short periods (maybe just within a boon, to begin with), and then if desired, gradually extending the duration of his enforced chastity as you explore how well it works for you.

## *Fantasy vs Reality*

If your slave does express a desire for device-based chastity, then the weirdness of his fantasies might surprise you. He might hope for extremely cruel treatment — a common male fantasy is to be kept locked up for months or years, perhaps being allowed an orgasm on his birthday, or even never at all. This is unlikely to mesh with your own desires, which presumably include seeing his penis and maybe even enjoying it from time to time! Also, there may be a health risk associated with such an extended period of chastity, since regular ejaculation can apparently protect against prostate problems in later life.

Another common male chastity fantasy involves close and regular supervision by the keyholder: if the device is the only thing keeping him chaste, and if you're the only person who can unlock it, then your supervision (read: your erotic attention) will be required whenever he must remove it for reasons of hygiene, to check for chafing, or for any other reason.

You should be clear in your own mind about how far you are prepared to go in catering to such fantasies, bearing in mind that you can respect and even indulge his fantasy without fulfilling every detail; telling him what he needs to hear during a boon (and acting part of it out) doesn't mean you have to go to the extremes that he thinks he wants.

Another consideration is that following an extended period of chastity, pent-up arousal may leave your slave's penis so hyper-sensitive that the intense stimulation of intercourse leads to him ejaculating before you are ready. Because of this, a strong emphasis on male chastity may be more suitable if you are happy to enjoy your slave in other ways, or you don't mind planning ahead to ensure he isn't too much on a "hair trigger" when you're looking for some staying power. Giving him a "ruined orgasm" (see page 85) can also be a way to help him recover quickly and then last longer.

## *Broaching the Subject*

It is quite possible that your slave will broach the subject of male chastity to you. If so, this chapter will have given the background information you need to decide whether you wish to play in this way, and if so how much control you're prepared to take and what kinds of rules you wish to use.

If you decide to take control of his orgasms without him having suggested it first, then you're going to have to take the lead. One way to begin is tell him, when he would normally expect to have an orgasm, that you want him to "wait until tomorrow", or even, "wait until next time" — perhaps informing him that you're changing things around so that you get an extra orgasm instead.

Then, before he's allowed release the next day (assuming he *is* to be allowed release), make sure he is in no doubt about how turned on you were at the thought of him being frustrated all night.

Your boons are already based on your pleasure and his sacrifice, and introducing an element of honor chastity is a natural extension of that. It can be a fun way of expressing your dominance occasionally, even if you don't wish to make orgasm control a major part of the routine you have with your slave.

## *Teasing and Denial*

Your slave will almost certainly not respond well if you lock him into a chastity device, or forbid him to masturbate, and consider that the end of the matter. He wants you to be an active and enthusiastic owner of his penis, to enjoy the control that you have, and even to flaunt your power over him. If none of those things interest you, this is probably not an aspect of female dominance that will work for you — and there's no reason it should work for everyone.

Your active participation is doubly important with device-based chastity because whatever interaction you offer him, will be his only erotic outlet.

The things he is hoping for may include:

- To have you take strict control over his opportunities for sexual pleasure, to reach orgasm, and even to have an erection (if you are using a chastity device).

- To have you acknowledge and enjoy your control/ownership, including by taking advantage of his restrained state by teasing him verbally and/or physically.

- To mercilessly refuse him orgasms, even when he is desperate for release.

- To be allowed the opportunity to enjoy giving you orgasms, in place of the orgasms he might otherwise have enjoyed himself.

- To receive *some* sexual stimulation even if he's not allowed to climax. If he's locked in, this might represent being unlocked while you tease his penis beyond what he can endure (or simply for a certain period of time or a number of strokes) before re-locking him. With the honor method, you could just manually tease him until he's groaning with frustration, and then tell him to put his pants back on.

- To have the opportunity for an occasional orgasm at your discretion — assuming he works hard enough at pleasing you.

- Possibly, to be forcibly subjected to extreme/permanent forms of chastity; this may be fine as a fantasy or as a role-play scenario, but I cannot recommend it in practice.

- Possibly, to explore through fantasy and role-play other scenarios related to the loss of male status associated with surrendering control of the penis, such as cuckolding, public exposure, enforced cross-dressing, or emasculation — all of which are quite common sexual fantasies, even if they will seem extreme to many.

## *Ruined Orgasms*

A "ruined orgasm" is an orgasm that is interrupted before it becomes fully satisfying. You can use it as a punishment or as an occasional, unexpected way of demonstrating your control. If your slave gets off on the sensations and psychological impact of being subjected to this treatment, then you might even view it as a reward.

The best time to administer a ruined orgasm is following an extended period of chastity, when he is intensely sensitive and desperate for release. There are several methods of inflicting a ruined orgasm, but this one is suitable for beginners:

Unless you are sure you can trust him not to "take over" at the critical moment, start by securing his hands. Apply lubrication to your fingers and then stroke him lightly, applying the minimum movement and friction needed to push him to the edge of climax. Depending on your man, you may be able to achieve this by rubbing the shaft of his penis (just below the head) between thumb and forefinger, or by lightly pinching his frenulum (the sensitive area on the underside of his penis, just below the head) and rapidly "twiddling it". If this level of stimulation doesn't get him there, grasp him with your circled, lubricated thumb and forefinger (don't use your other fingers), just below the head of his penis, and rub up and down.

Avoid stimulating the whole length of his penis, since that risks pushing your slave into a "normal" orgasm such as he would get from the deep thrusts of intercourse. Despite the unorthodox stimulation, his frustration should mean that it won't take much to bring him to the brink.

The instant he is over that brink, stop all stimulation immediately. If you get the timing right, he will have a ruined orgasm — his ejaculation will be muted, and his sense of pleasure and release will be far from what a normal orgasm would have offered.

If you get the timing wrong, then either he will not ejaculate at all (in which case you are free to continue teasing him, if you wish) or he may have a full orgasm. An advantage of springing a ruined orgasm as a surprise, is that he won't know what you intended in the first place. On the other hand, if you did tell him his orgasm would be ruined, then the fact that he went ahead and had one anyway (even if not entirely his fault), may well be grounds for punishment...

Another possibility for ruined orgasms comes from what many would see as a shortcoming of open cage/tube style chastity devices. If your slave is locked in such a device for a long period, he can become so frustrated and aroused, and his body so insistent on producing an erection, that the flesh of his penis presses through the cage openings. Stroking this flesh can then lead to an orgasm that is ruined by his inability to get properly erect, by the limited stimulation possible, and perhaps because of the squeezing/constricting effect of the tight tube.

This can offer your slave a way to cheat, but it also offers you a sex toy and a no-brainer way of giving him a ruined orgasm. Just keep him locked in, use plenty of lube, and masturbate him until he produces whatever climax and ejaculation is possible while constrained inside the device. Stop all stimulation as soon as he reaches the point of no return.

Your ability to ruin your slave's orgasms is a potent demonstration of his powerlessness and your control, and it might be that he really gets off on this. If so, then the existence of ruined orgasms can add to the mind blowingness of his real orgasms, if you offer him a judicious, teasing reminder of your power at the critical moment.

## Orgasm on Command

Some people hold that the most perfect form of orgasm control is where the submissive learns to climax when ordered to do so, requiring no stimulation except for that verbal command. This is unlikely to be achievable outside of fantasy, but it can be possible, with training and practice, to command an orgasm and to have your slave deliver one.

You might wonder why anyone would need to be told to have an orgasm, since men are usually so eager for sexual pleasure and release, but...

- a chastity-minded slave might prefer not to have an orgasm *right now*, since the long-term turn-on of remaining submissively pure could be more important to him than the momentary satisfaction of release.

- even a slave who wants an orgasm, might wish to control the timing. If nothing else, if an orgasm is on the cards for him then presumably he's engaged in sex with you (or at least enjoying your sexual attention). Surrendering to an orgasm too soon means cutting that pleasure short.

The kind of forced orgasm I'm discussing here is not the same as a ruined orgasm, even though ruined orgasms are usually forced. Nor is it about having intercourse (or otherwise stimulating him) with the intention of continuing until he climaxes.

An "orgasm on command" happens according to your schedule, and is fully satisfying for your slave — and to you as well, if you enjoy watching him perform at your command.

The goal is to make him delay his orgasm until you are ready, and then to climax as soon as possible once you give the word. Since you'll be busy stimulating him during the waiting part, this will take a lot of self-control on his part; he'll need your help and patience in order to learn it. What *you* will need to know are:

- exactly how his pre-orgasmic responses develop as you stimulate him, so that you can judge where he is, and tell when he is about to climax.

- what his "hot-buttons" are, so that you can physically or verbally push them and thus tip him over the edge.

Begin by taking him almost all the way to orgasm. Then, order him to come. Use the same commanding tone and the same form of words each time; the power of ritual will become part of what propels him along the required path.

Once you've given the command, trigger his orgasm by pushing the "hot buttons" that you know work for him. His hot-buttons might include the way you stimulate his penis or some other physical act, or it could be something you say — anything that you know plays powerfully to his personal kinks or fetishes, and that will kick him past the point of no return. Once he's ejaculated, let him know how pleased you are that he's obeyed you so well.

If you sense that he is coming too early, give the command immediately and go through the procedure; save any discussion of what went wrong for the aftercare phase. This is a learning process for both of you and there's always a next time. Bear in mind that:

- you can easily do things to force a climax before you've commanded it. This will usually be less rewarding than pushing him to the edge, and then enjoying his responses as he desperately tries to resist.
- if he's tired or sexually sated, he might have the opposite problem: inability to deliver an orgasm promptly in response to your command. This will usually be a physical issue that will resolve itself with rest and abstinence.
- the fullness of his bladder can affect his responsiveness; the pressure will make it harder for him to delay, but easier for him to deliver when you give the word.
- the pressure of a hinged[1] or flexible cock ring (one that fits over both penis and scrotum, sitting snugly against his body) can have a similar effect. If you own a tube-based chastity device that locks to him with a hinged ring (or even an old hair scrunchy) then you already have something suitable.

Over time, as he learns better control and as the ritual aspect of your control grows in power, you can gradually rely more on your command, and less on other button-pushing, to trigger his orgasm. If you like, test him with some gentle button-pushing *before* you give the command. Eventually, you may end up with your command itself becoming a major hot-button for him, perhaps even the only one you need.

1    Compared to a solid ring, a hinged or flexible ring is much safer because it can always be removed quickly. The risk is that a small, solid cock ring + large, erect penis = visit to the emergency room.

Please be aware that fine control over orgasm is not something that every man will be able to learn. If your slave simply cannot hold back until you tell him to climax, or if he cannot respond promptly to your command, then don't worry — there are plenty of other ways for you to have dominant, orgasm-controlling fun with him.

## Enforcement of Chastity

If you're using honor-based chastity, then enforcement can only come from you. If you're using device-based chastity, enforcement comes from the lockable device itself ... *in theory.*

In practice, even a well-designed chastity device from a reputable maker may not always be escape proof. It may be possible for him to pull out of a cage/tube device sufficiently to have an orgasm (and then to re-insert himself). And as mentioned above, a long period in chastity may leave him in such a hair-trigger state that he can manage a ruined orgasm without getting out of the device at all.

So, if you want to be sure he's not cheating, you need a way to tell when he's recently had an orgasm.

(If you're thinking that your slave wouldn't dare lie to you, or even disobey you in the first place, then you might well be right (or you might not be!). It doesn't matter. Female dominance is most potent when it's imposed on a strong (though submissive) male, not when it's meekly accepted by a milksop. More than that, it needs to be *seen* to be imposed. Otherwise, there would be no point in having Boons, Quests, Punishments, Rituals, or any of the other things discussed in this book; you'd just tell your man what you wanted, and he would just do it, and you'd both save a lot of time ... and have a lot less fun together).

The first sign that he has cheated after a lengthy period in chastity, will be a change in his behavior. Where previously he was naturally attentive and eager to please, his attentiveness may now appear forced or rehearsed. Perhaps he'll seem unexpectedly relaxed, or display sudden symptoms of post-orgasm male grumpiness — if you've been with your slave for a while, you'll know how he responds.

Another way to tell whether he's recently had an orgasm, is to become familiar with his physical responses at different stages: an hour after he's had an orgasm, for example, or the next morning, or twenty-four hours later. How quickly does he become erect when you touch or squeeze him? How hard is he? What's his breathing like? Is his body quivering with frustrated desperation? Or does he seem strangely relaxed? If you allow him an orgasm (or a ruined orgasm) after a period of chastity, how long before he recovers?

His responses and recovery when frustrated will be strikingly different from the norm, and with experience you can use this to judge how honest he's being. Keeping him on the straight-and-narrow also provides the perfect excuse for you to have regular teasing sessions with him — which will be pleasurable for him as well, and so an extra motivation to remain true.

If you find that your slave has cheated, then you must take it seriously. Even if he denies it, his punishment is always at your discretion; he will not want you to "let him off" simply because he claims to have done nothing wrong. The more certain you are that he has cheated, the less inclined you should be to inflict punishments that he might confuse with a reward (such as being sentenced to a further period in chastity, which is pointless anyway, if he's going to cheat).

So, to punish cheating, choose something that doesn't turn him on. Even the most masochistic slave is unlikely to be aroused by a cold shower, or by being made to sit alone to compose a letter of apology. Remember to remove any erotic rituals that you might normally use to spice up his punishments.

Of course, the ultimate punishment is to withdraw the boon of controlling his orgasms, or at least to suspend it until he can prove himself (perhaps through a suitable period of honor-chastity). At the end of the day, if he can't honor you by complying with your control, there is no reason for you to honor him by continuing to provide it.

# *Reflecting on Orgasm Control*

This section is for you to examine your feelings about taking control of your slave's orgasms, and various issues that can arise from that.

| | |
|---|---|
| I should be the only source of erotic fulfilment that my slave needs | Yes ☐ <br> No ☐ |
| When my slave is sexually frustrated, I enjoy it | Yes ☐ <br> No ☐ |
| I think my slave is self-disciplined enough to succeed with "honor chastity" | Yes ☐ <br> No ☐ |
| I would like my slave to be more attentive to me | Yes ☐ <br> No ☐ |
| I would like my slave to be permanently aroused around me | Yes ☐ <br> No ☐ |
| The idea of having my slave discreetly under lock-and-key appeals to me | Yes ☐ <br> No ☐ |
| I am entitled to receive more orgasms than my slave | Yes ☐ <br> No ☐ |

*(if "Yes" above, I should receive around _____ for each one of his)*

| | |
|---|---|
| My slave should earn his orgasms | Yes ☐ <br> No ☐ |

Unauthorized orgasms for my slave should be discouraged or punished

Yes ☐
No ☐

How I would feel about restricting my slave's orgasms

Aroused ☐
Intrigued ☐
Pragmatic ☐
Accepting ☐
Justified ☐
Embarrassed ☐
Disturbed ☐
Puzzled ☐

Three possible results of limiting my slave's orgasms and controlling when he has them, that would benefit me:

1. _____

2. _____

3. _____

Three possible results of limiting my slave's orgasms and controlling when he has them, that would trouble or inconvenience me:

1. _____

2. _____

3. _____

Ruined orgasms should be a possibility for my slave — Yes ☐ No ☐

How I would feel about ruining my slave's orgasms

Aroused ☐
Intrigued ☐
Pragmatic ☐
Accepting ☐
Justified ☐
Embarrassed ☐
Disturbed ☐
Puzzled ☐

When I consider ruining my slave's orgasms, I feel:

_____

_____

_____

_____

_____

_____

_____

94

Forced orgasms (on command) should be a possibility for my slave — Yes ☐ No ☐

How I would feel about commanding my slave's orgasms — Aroused ☐ Intrigued ☐ Pragmatic ☐ Accepting ☐ Justified ☐ Embarrassed ☐ Disturbed ☐ Puzzled ☐

When I consider commanding my slave's orgasms, I feel:

_____

_____

_____

_____

_____

_____

_____

Some "hot-button" issues that could push my slave into climax are:

_____

_____

_____

_____

_____

_____

_____

_____

_____

_____

_____

_____

# *Ten Basic Rules*

They have but few laws, and such is their constitution that they need not many.

— Sir Thomas More —
*Utopia*

1.  If you're not comfortable with something, it doesn't happen.

2.  His male submission is a desire; your female dominance is a boon.

3.  The boon of worship, may also be orgasmic to you.

4.  The boon of servitude, may also be useful to you.

5.  The boon of punishment, may also be satisfying to you.

6.  Each of your boons is a gift of your female erotic attention.

7.  He longs to know that you recognize and value his submission.

8.  Rituals can offer a short-cut to where you and he want to go.

9.  For maximum erotic tension, allow him enough time to *anticipate*.

10. For maximum erotic submission, control his orgasms.

*Also by Lucy Fairbourne*

*Male Chastity:*
*A Guide for Keyholders*

Printed in the USA
CPSIA information can be obtained
at www.ICGtesting.com
LVHW020831080124
768369LV00003B/121